911
EMERGENCY
HEALTH

NATURAL HEALTH
CONSULTANT

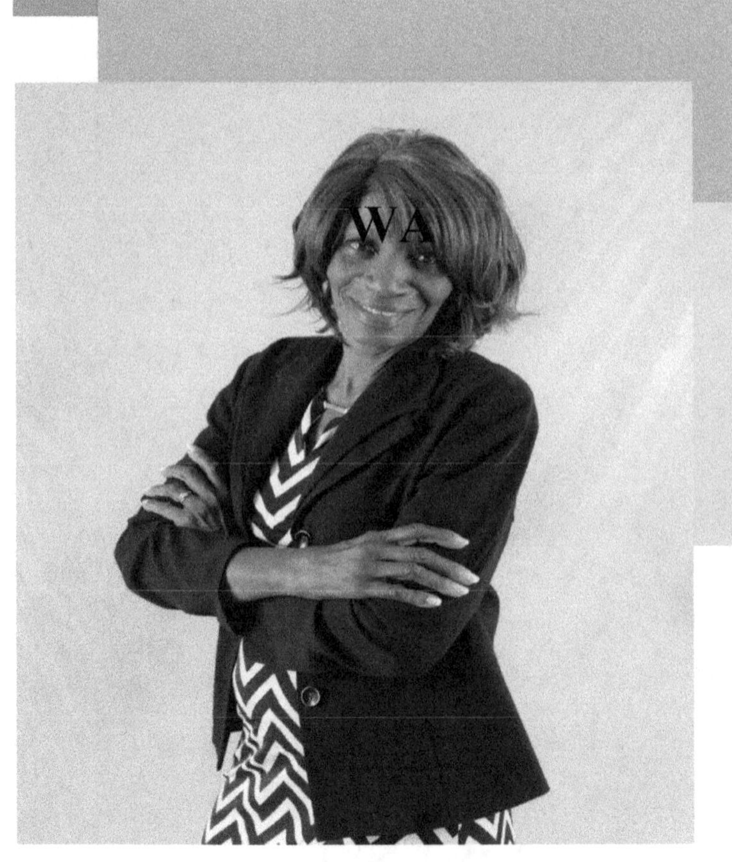

DR. WARDINE SAUNDERS

WARDINE SAUNDERS

Edition (1 of 3)

911 Emergency Health

What's your Emergency?

Fatigue, Allergies, Chronic Illnesses, Weight Loss, Arthritis, Diabetes, High Blood Cancer, Cholesterol, and Chronic Pain., etc.

You can make a copy and pass it

Content:

CREATION
WHY I WROTE THIS BOOK
911 HEALTH
DEDICATION
WEIGHT CHART I
AM UNIVERSITY
DR. SEBI EAT TO HEAL COME
BACK TO THE GARDEN 10—14
REVERSE YOUR ILLNESS CLEANSE
& DETOX
9 HERB TEA REVERSE!
REVERSE! 10-14 DAYS
NEW LIFE NO REFINED
FOODS PLANT FIBER

NO AMINAL FOODS NO
VEGETABLE OILS 10-
14 DAYS NUTRITION &
LIFE THE NEW YOU
LIFE STYLE CHANGE
FIGHT DESEASE

MEAT BASE DIET AMAZING BODY
BASIC DIET This what my JUICING
healthy look at
45 SUPER FOOD 70 a birthday on
LUNCH & DINNER February 25 .
SALTY FLAVORS
LINDER LARKINS 70 YRS My first self
HEALTH CONSUITANT publish Book.
PRAYERS FOR HEALTH Everyone should
PRE-ORDER BOOK do it.

CREATION

*All Scripture quotations, unless noted
otherwise; Hebrew Greek Key Study Bible;
Vines Dictionary of Bible Words; Webster's
Collegiate Dictionary. I will prove to you that
the Creator wanted us to use Herbs &
Veggies to drink and*
eat for meat, not animals at all.
Gen. 1:26,29; Ezekiel 47:12; Rev. 22:2.
Everyone has some type of body
problems, even if it's just a stomach ache.
The body needs attention too. Our body
respond when something is wrong inside.
This is the only way it can let us know
something's wrong. We will experience pain
or some type of abnormal feeling. Which
tells us something is wrong.

When our body wants to eat, It will make us
feel hungry. Sometimes we feel lazy,
irritable or miserable. Your body is always
talking to us, we need to watch what we put
in it. Our body is like electricity. It absorbs
everything that go in it. Thank God for the
doctors : Dr. David Servan, Dr Schreiber
and Dr. Neal Barnard, Dr. Sebi, just a few,
WHO HAVE TURN TO Naturopathy
Medicine, without doctors a lot of us would
have passed on already slowly. And some
of us will suffer and die from pharmaceutical
conventional medication slowly. So start
eating more fruits & veggies.

WHY DID I WRITE THIS BOOK

I'm on a mission to help as many people I can who wants Emergency Health! It's not about me but us, and whoever wants to live **a HEALTHY and ENERGETIC life, like me at 70,** I've seen too many of my friends pass-on at an early age from **High Blood pressure, Diabetes, different types of Cancer and Kidney problems**. I started selling herbal products 5 years ago and I have always been networking with others in the field of natural alternatives to create natural health products. When I went to a herbal tea party, it amazed me about all the benefits herbs did for the body. If you have any questions, feel free to contact me or go to my website and view natural products that are helping to enhance lives. Remember God

the Creator planted these herbs for the healing of the Nations **(Genesis 2:9; Ez. 47:12; Rev. 22:2)** because He knew we were going to get sick from all ***this junk and toxin** foods we absolve in our*

CONTINUE

My name is Wardine but most of my friends call me Zehira. My granddaughter named me Herbie because whenever they came to me with health issues like cramps, headaches, coughs, colds and pain I would prescribe an herb remedy. When they started to heal, feel better and return to good health, they don't laugh at me anymore. Now, they come to me and ask me for advice for teas and herbal remedies. For me personally, I started drinking tea for menopause and it worked. Now I start drinking different teas for many different things (ailments). I don't take no prescribed medications, this is my choice. This year so far, my physical health has been really good which I attribute to herbs and veggies and fruits. I feel truly blessed to have 5 children, 18 grand children, 4 great grands and I'm only 70 years young and I feel

great! started selling herbal products over10 years ago. *I have enroll in a School of natural health Consultant Now The University of I AM gave me a Doctors award*

911 EMERGENCY HEALTH

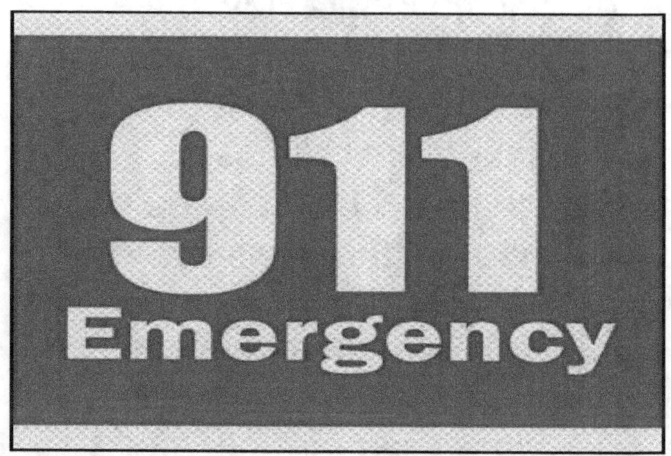

Why I say Emergency, because it means we need help right now!
Also mean a serious unexpected and often dangerous situation inquiring immediate action. Quick response in an emergency could be a lifesaver. A person with a medical condition requiring immediate treatment. When you have any of these conditions, it require emergency attention! Heart Disease, High Blood Pressure, Diabetes, Cancer, Chronic Pain, Blood Clots, and many

more; Call 911 Emergency Health! There are licensed Naturopathy Physicians trained in clinical nutrition, acupuncture, homeopathic, botanical medicine, psychology, and counseling to encourage you to make lifestyle changes and support your personal health.

DEDICATION

I give all praises, worship and honor to Almighty God Creator, Who has giving me the inspiration to *write this book. It is a blessing for*
me and it will be for you too. The Creator created us and gave us directions on how to take care of our body, Genesis 1:29; read it and learn what I saw.

To my memory of darling mother, who is the essence of love, who has always been my personal source of encouragement and inspiration, and passionate commitment to excellence in leadership. Suffered with colon cancer.

To my daughters and son, Abigail, Nita, Patricia, Lela and Isaac, who I love dearly. They continue to provide incentive for the exercise and development of my leadership potential success and purpose. And I hope I have inspired someone else along the way.

And to all the millions of great men and women who presently occupy the womb of the mothers, their destiny.

And to all the third world peoples around the world whose potentate were and in some cases still are oppressed and suppressed by the opinions and judgments of others. And to all the aspiring leaders researching on information about herbs and nutrition benefits for our health.

CHECK YOUR WEIGHT CHART MEASURMENT

IDEAL
4' 10" 91—105 5' 7" 121—140 4'
11" 94—109 5' 0" 100—116 5' 0"
97—112 5' 9" 128—149 5' 1" 100—
116 5' 10" 132—153 5' 2" 104– 120
5' 11" 136—157 5' 3" 107—124 6'
0" 140—162 5' 4" 110—128 6' 1"
144—166 5' 5" 114—132 6' 2"
148—171 5' 6" 118—136 6' 3"
152—176

GOOD
4' 10" 105—119 5' 7" 140—159 4'

11" 109—124 5' 8" 144—164 5' 0"

112—128 5' 9" 149—169 5' 1"

116—132 5' 10" 153—174 5' 2"

120—136 6' 0" 157—179 5' 3"

124—141 6' 1" 162—184 5' 4"

128—150 6' 2" 166—189 5' 5"

132—155 6' 3" 176—200

IDEAL—GOOD—OVER WEIGHT—OBESE

OVER WEIGHT
4' 10" 105—143 5' 7" 159—191 4'
11" 124—148 5' 8" 164—197 5' 0"
128—153 5' 9" 169—203 5' 1"
132—158 5' 10" 174—209 5' 2"
136—164 5' 11" 179—215 5' 3"
141—169 6' 0" 184—221 5' 4"
145—174 6' 1" 189—227 5' 5"
150—180 6' 2" 194—233 5' 6"
155—186 6' 3" 200—240

OBESE
4' 10" 143 + 5' 7" 191 + 4'
11" 148 + 5' 8 197 + 5' 0"
153 + 5' 9" 203 + 5' 1" 158 +
5' 10" 209 + 5' 2" 164 + 5'
11" 215 + 5' 3" 169 + 6' 0"
221 + 5' 4" 174 + 6' 3" 227 +
5' 5" 180 + 6' 2" 233 + 5' 6"
186 + 6' 3" 240 +

ROSE WALKER THE OWNER OF I AM

UNIVERSITY Presented me with this

certificate at the WOMEN OF WISDOM

EVENT

**The Honorary Doctor Of Humane Letter
I have been helping healing the community
with Herbs and Nutrition for over 20 years.
I'm also studying at Stratford Career Institute
to be a Natural Health Consultant this year.**

**These Are Doctors And Practitionals In
The US:
Allopathic (Western Medicine)
Ayurvedic Medicine (Balance with
Nature) Chiropractic (Spine, Back Bone
Health) Environmental medicine
(Allergens & Chemical Toxics)
Herbalism (Plant Based Substances) Holistic
Dentistry (No Silver Filling) Homeopathy
(Stimulate Immune System) Midwifery
(Overseeing The Birth of Children)
Naturopathic Medicine (Restore Body To
Heal Itself)
Osteopathic Medicine (Treatment of
Body Joints)**

"EAT TO HEAL YOUR BODY"
Dr. Sebi Book—Eat To Heal

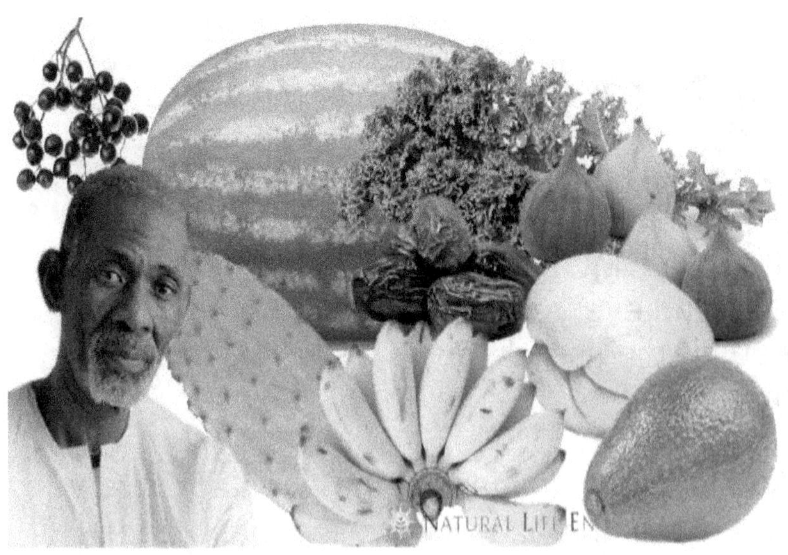

Dr. Sebi healed Aids, Cancer and the Blind.
He has a lot of information on youtube.

WATERMELON, COCONUT, KALE, CALALOO,
SPINACH, AVOCADO, GREEN BANANAS,
GARBANZO BEANS, CATUS FLOWER & LEAF,
LETTUCE EXCEPT ICEBERG, CUCUMBER,
SQUASH, (Mexican) , SEA VEGIES, CHERRY
OR PLUM TOMATOES, ZUCCHINI,
WATERCRESS, & BELL PEPPERS.
Delicious Fruits:

APPLES, CHERRIES, CURRANTS, DATES,
FIGS, GRAPES SEEDED, LIMES,ORANGE
(Seville or sour), MANGO, MELONS SEEDED,
PAPAYAS, PEACHES, PEAR, PLUMS, PRUNES,
RAISINS (seeded), SOFT JELLY COCONUTS,
SOURSOPS & TAMARINE.

COME BACK TO THE GARDEN OF HEALING
(GOD'S WORDS: Gen. 2:29, Ez. 47:12; Rev. 22:2

The Creator's Directions for the body:
"And God said. See, I have given you every plant yielding seed (not fruit without seeds, they are GMO) that is on the face of all the land and every tree in which is the fruit of the tree yielding seed; to you it shall be for meat." (no animal)

And to all the animals on the earth and every bird of the air and to everything that creeps on the ground, to everything in which there is the breath life I have given every green plant for food. And it was so. (Genesis 1:29) Honor your father and mother. Then you will live a long full life in the land the Lord your God is giving you! (Exodus 20:12) If you not living a long fulfilled life in good health, you are not obeying God's words. **Obey and live long healthy life!**

For Questions: 954-709-7584

Email Me:
miraclehealing7@yahoo.com

Information about products How to do juice your fruit & veggies

10-14 DAYS REVERSE YOUR
ILNESS (HEALTH)

Creator means, a person who bring something in existence, like all the stuff we have in our possession. They were created by someone and they put directions with it. Therefore our Creator Who is God gave us directions to follow too: we over looked our instruction and went with man's directions for our body. This is why we have all this different sickness because of it. If you did not create something, you are not suppose to try to figure how you think it is suppose to work, most likely you are going to make a mistake on the directions. We was not created to be sick, I don't see all the sickness I hear about in the Bible. When we become sick, we are in violation of our Creator's directions; no exceptions it's true.

Gen. 2:9; Ezekiel 47:12; Rev. 22:2. DOCTORS AND

PRACTITIONALS IN THE U.S:

Allopathic (Western medicine)
Ayurvedic Medicine (Balance with Nature)
Herbalism / Lifestyle & dietary Change. Allopathy / pharmaceutical *Chiropractic (Spine, Back bone health) Herbalism (Plant-based Holistic Dentistry (No Midwifery (Overseeing the Naturopathic Medicine (itself) Natural Medicine Osteopathic Medicine (Treatment*

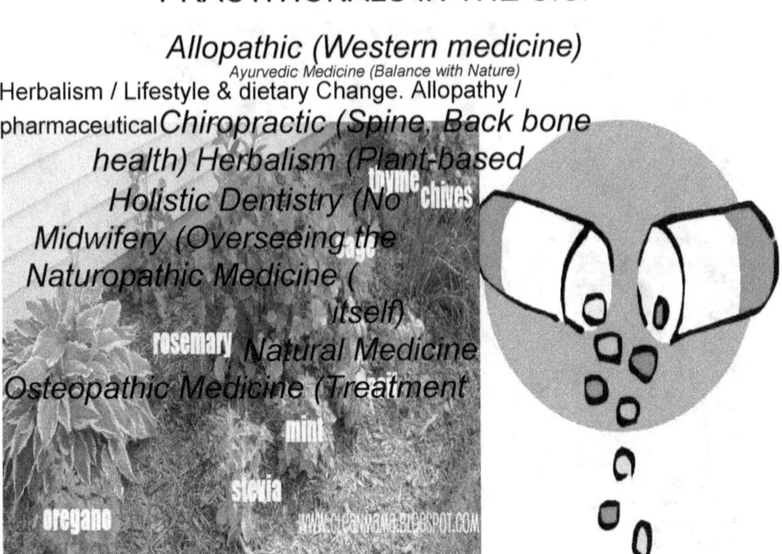

FIRST THING: CLEANSE AND DETOX WITH YOUR CHOICE OF TEAS.

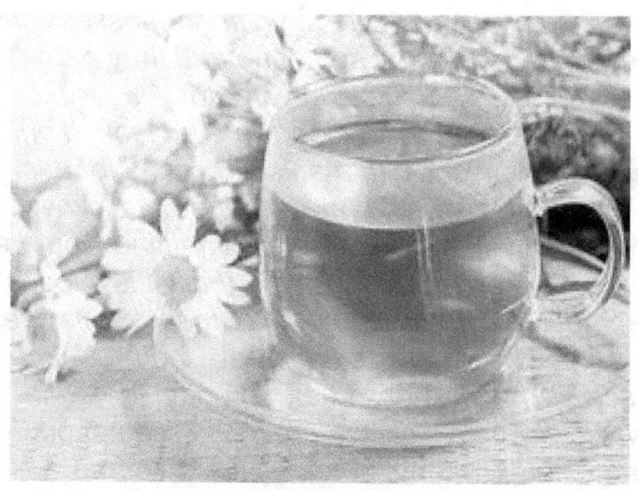

**Organic Chamomile
Tea
And 12 Herb Tea
Cleanse and Detox**

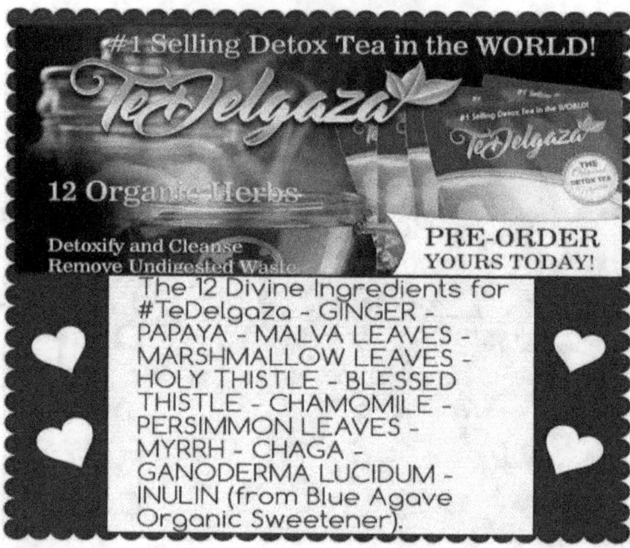

9 ORGANIC HERB TEA

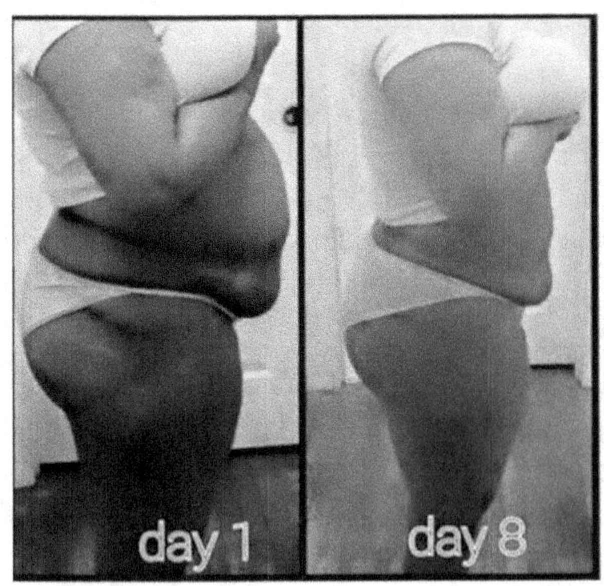

Drink 2 cups of tea a day...

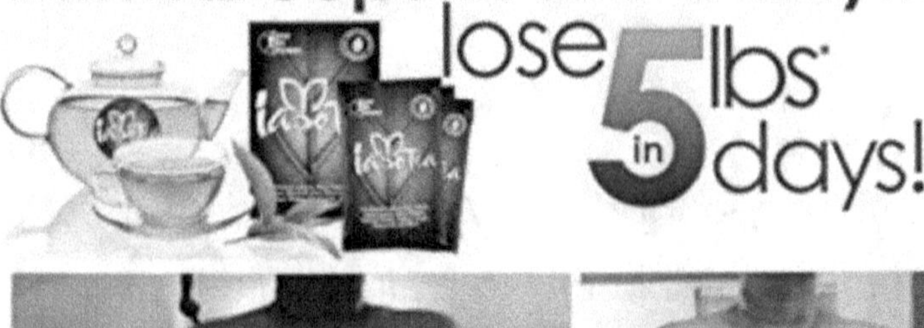

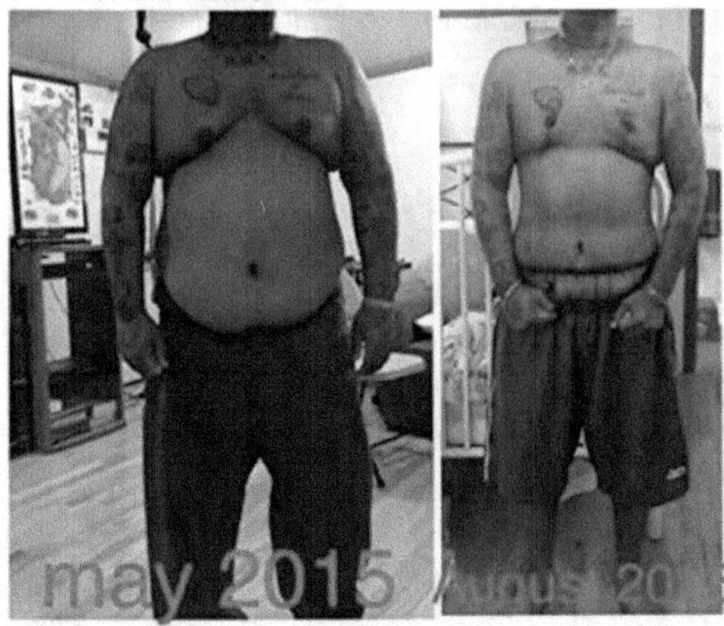

REVERSE! REVERSE MY HEALTH!!!

The REVERSE Diet is uncompromising and strict adherence to it won't be possible for many. If that is the case for you, it should be thought of as an ideal diet—something strive for—because the closer you followed to the letter, it works and works wonders. The REVERSE Diet is uncompromising and strict adherence to it won't be possible for many. If that is the case for you, it should be thought of as an ideal diet—something strive for— because the closer you followed to the letter, it works and works wonders.

No Refined foods No Animal foods (Meats) No Vegetable oil No Dairy, Milk, Butter, Cheese And Exercise.

The following sections provide an

<u>Explanation.</u>

14 DAYS TO A NEW YOU

When we say " 14 days to a new you!" we're not talking about JUST losing pounds in days, but changing your tastes for food in just 2 weeks. That's how long it takes most people to make a complete switch in their taste buds. The problem is that we have lost our taste for natural foods because most of the food we eat today is smothered **with salt, fat, sweets and chemicals.** As a result, our taste buds has become warped as we crave the "highs" of sugar, fat and salt that have become a standard part of the typical

American diet. In other words, **our taste buds are really driving our diseases**.

Your taste for food will change with this new way of eating and you will find you prefer the cleaner taste of natural foods. After eating this way, you'll find that the high fat foods will taste greasy. Many people have told me that when they do eat high-fat foods, their entire system slows down and they feel sluggish.

Stick to the REVERSE Diet for 14 days and you're find you won't want to go back to the heavy, calorie -dense foods you've been eating. In just 14 days, your taste will change, You're be on your way to permanent **WEIGHT loss** and a health change, you're be feeling better to boot!

NO REFINED FOODS

Unhealthy food is available everywhere all the time, like never before in history. Gas station, drug stores, schools… Dr. Kelly D. Brownell, Yale University.

Refined foods are plant foods that have been **denatured and stripped of their fiber, vitamins, minerals, antioxidants and other nutrients**. These foods are lifeless imitations of the vibrant products found in
nature. They are devoid of any nutritional value and are usually transformed into dull, man-made food stuffs that do not satisfy hunger, wreak
havoc on your health and generally don't require teeth to eat them.
Sadly, about half of the total calories in a typical American diet come from refined foods.

Refined foods are simple **carbohydrates such as white flour, wheat flour, refined sugar, pastries, white semolina, white bread, white rice, french fries, chips of any variety, cakes, soft drinks and similar junk foods.** You know the foods I'm talking about—foods that have been transformed from

their natural state into man-made products.
The only rice product allowed are whole brown rice. Always use whole- wheat pastas, whole wheat or whole grain breads because they kept their fiber on the way to the grocery store. With grain products, the **first ingredient should always have the word "whole"** in it, sprouted wheat or organic rolled oats. Don't let the words **"hearty wheat, "stone wheat," or multigrain on the package fool you.**

Plant fiber does a number of miraculous things for your health, but one thing it does best is remove toxic substances from your body so you can flush them down the toilet.
Fiber even removes heavy metals such as mercury, which you probably have in your body as a result of eating fish or farm animals that were fed fish meal. Fiber also removes cholesterol—the reason a fiber rich—diet will lower your cholesterol. In addition, fiber bind sex hormones, such as estrogen, and removes them from your body. **In the case of estrogen, American women have very high levels of estrogen due not only to our high-fat diet, but also due the lack of fiber in our diets.**

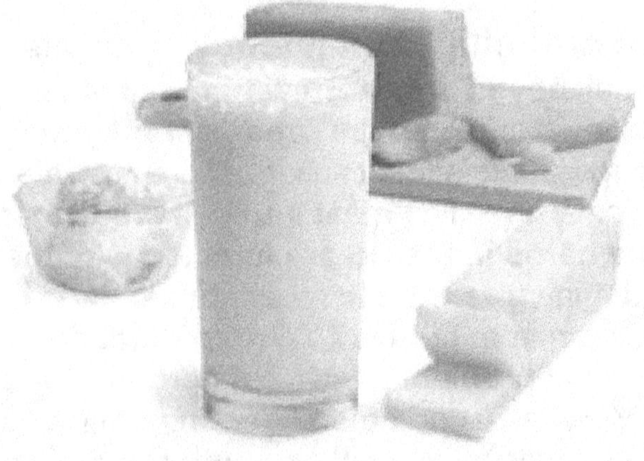

All Dairy products has estrogen . (Fattening) That makes us gain weight. Milk, Cheese, Yogurt, eggs and lots more.

NO ANIMAL FOODS

The only thing you'll miss from eating animal foods is the saturated fat, cholesterol and animal proteins— as well as the diseases these ingredients bring to your body. The more you eat whole plant foods, the less likely you will gain weight. In a recent multi-nation study, it was found that without exception, the thinnest people ate a complex carbohydrate diet, while the fattest people ate a meat base diet.

Eliminating meat from your diet is essential if you want to achieve your ideal weight, reverse heart disease and protect yourself against cancers and our major degenerative diseases.

With stunning consistency, **nutrients from all animal foods grew tumors, while nutrients from all plant foods shrank tumors.** With respect to some cancers, there is a little known problem with eating **meat and dairy: 89% percent of the herds in the US are infected with the leukemia virus, which cause leukemia and lymphomas in people.. This isn't just an American problem as 84% of herbs in Argentina and 70% in Canada also have the bovine leukemia virus, as well as in other meat eating countries.**

Each year about 30,000 new cases of leukemia and 70,000 new cases of lymphoma occur for unknown reasons in the US, many are caused by bovine. The best way to protect yourself against this virus, is to avoid meat and dairy products. Change your eating habit as it's been shown to greatly reduce your risk of being infected.

NO VEGETABLE OILS

Strictly speaking, vegetable oils are part of the Refined Foods group because they contain no fiber, they're devoid of nutrients and they're 100% fat.

Although I say vegetable oils, because these are what are ok consumed, mean any oils (e.g., nut oils, coconut oil, olive oil etc.). **Omega—**3 in vegetable oil are highly
unstable and tend to decompose and unleash free radicals and cause damage to cells. **Vegetable oils** has also been implicated in several different studies with **cancers and polyunsaturated fat** turn out to be the strongest promoter of **skin cancers of all the foodstuff we eat.** Vegetable oils also supports the immune system and actually promote the spread of cancers. Don't cook with olive and other oils they will bankrupt foods that have little nutritional value.

Instead of using vegetable oils for cooking, cook at lower temperatures and use water to make your own broth– are use the substitutes below:

Oil substitutes for Sauteing: Apple juice, Sherry, Vegetable stock, Vinegars, Wine and Beer., If you not trying to lose weight, coconut oil.

Oil substitutes in baked good: Applesauce,
Pureed bananas, Pureed stewed prunes.

For salads choose a dressing without oil. A vinegar based dressing, such as: Balsamic or Brown rice seasoned vinegar dressing. Or try citrus juices in place of salad dressing. without oil.

10– 14 DAYS TO A NEW YOU

Now after all these negative "NO's",
you're probably thinking I'm crazy for also saying "No
Exceptions" because everyone is going to have some
exceptions in our world of plentiful temptations. If you
are simply trying to lose weight, as opposed to
reversing a disease, then I would say you could apple
a "99 percent" Nutrition rule.

Roger Ebert the film critic, lost 89 pounds and
described rare exception like this: I agree with
McDonald that a visit can be part of a responsible
nutritional approach. That's way I've dined there twice
in last 17 months.

EXERCISE
Exercise is an essential part of the REVERSE Diet.
Exercise also speeds the passage of carcinogens and
toxins from the body and recent studies have shown
that exercise keeps your brain as fit as your body,
particularly as you age. In other words, exercise will not
only make you feel fit and improve your appearance,
but it will prevent a wide range of diseases.

ESSENTIAL DIETARY GUIDELINES
Here are a few simple keys to the Nutrition Diet:

The #1 Golden Rule: Always eat foods as close to
their natural state as possible. Eat whole foods that
come in their natural packages and avoid foods that
come in cans, unless they are fresh-frozen. Some of
the sample menus will contain items that are
canned. This is for convenience.

NUTRITION AND LIFESTYLE

Always eat Whole foods: In package goods, look for the words "whole" "sprouted" wheat" or "organic rolled oats". Always eat whole-wheat pastas or whole wheat breads. Make sure the label says whole wheat, not wheat flour. Don't let the words "hearty wheat," stoned wheat," or multigrain" on the package fool you. Such ingredients are made from refined white flour and there's no difference between white flour and wheat flour. Wheat flour has some caramel coloring and sounds healthier, but it's not.

Eat a wide variety of colorful foods:
Always eat a wide variety of foods because each food has it's own special health benefits and disease fighting profiles-and they work as a team, complimenting, reinforcing and magnifying each other benefits. This is the new math of cancer prevention and eating a variety of foods actually multiplies cancer-fighting and cardiovascular benefits because they work together synergistically. So make sure your plate is full of different colors– the deeper and darker the colors, the more cancer fighting nutrients.

Uncooked Food: Eat at least half of your food uncooked.
The more uncooked food, the better, In general, cooked or processed foods contain fewer phytochemicals and antioxidants than fresh and uncooked foods.

10-14 DAYS TO A NEW YOU

Kale, Arugula, Watercress and other vegetables such as , , brussels sprouts, radishes, and are the best sources of a powerful anti -cancer nutrient called suforaphane. Steaming is the best way to cook vegetables. Try to eat your food plain or with herbs and spices.

A Salad Is An Ideal Meal: If you find salad takes too much time to prepare, simple stop by your local salad bar, be it in a restaurant or supermarket-but bring your own salad dressing, or use vinegar without oil. If you use slice beets, the juice from them can serve a delicious salad.

Chew your food thoroughly: The ideal behind reversing disease with nutrition is to give your body a concentrated boost of nutrients. The key to this is the ability to fully digest the foods you are eating, in order to get the most nutrients from them. This is where the
enzymes come into play because enzymes help your body fully digest food. **Your food should be close to liquid before you swallow it, you should drink your food.**

Never cook with salt: Natural plant food contain all the sodium you'll ever need. People like to say that salt brings out the favor in food. Nonsense! All it does is give food a salty taste and camouflage the real taste of the
food, while promoting blood clotting and high blood pressure. **Learn to use spices and herbs, instead of salt, those that have High Blood, to flavor your food. Try Mrs. Dash or Salt-Free Spike or sea salt with iron.**

LIFE STYLE CHANGE

Snacking: Snacking in-between meals is not bad. It all depends on what you eat. Avoid package "snack" Always eat whole plant foods, such as fruit or vegetables. Fruits are the best snacks.

Beverages: Pure water should always be the beverage of choice. Any beverage containing any kind of sweetener is off limits. Any beverage containing a stimulant, such as caffeine once a day if you must have coffee, should be avoided. Fruit juices are fine as long as they are unsweetened and contain the fiber or pulp from the whole fruit. Drink as much water you are comfortable with. If you are trying to loss weight fast. Look at Accelerating weight loss.

Eating out: Ethnic restaurants usually have the best food choices, but ask them to leave out the bad stuff following the **REVERSE Diet** rules. Simply you don't eat meat and dairy and ask them to prepare a vegetable plate for you.
First of all everyone eats plant foods. Rice, potatoes, lettuce, cherry tomatoes, fruits, bread and so forth are all part of our diets and we all eat a wider range of plant foods than they realize. Just too little of them.
All you do is substitute that slice of steak or

chicken on your plate with more plant foods.

I cook red beans and green frozen

beans for protein too.

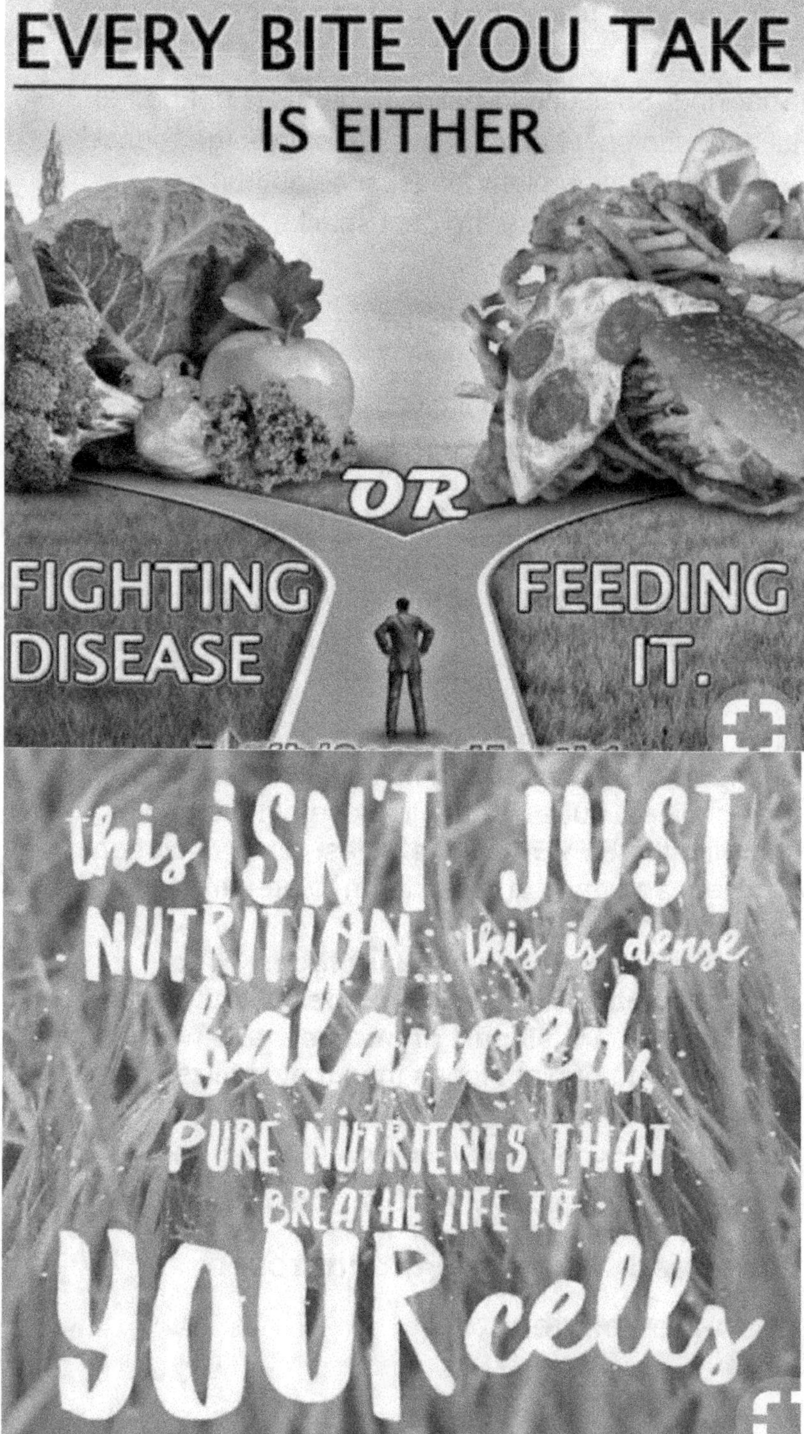
EVERY BITE YOU TAKE
IS EITHER
OR
FIGHTING DISEASE
FEEDING IT.
this ISN'T JUST NUTRITION... this is dense, balanced, PURE NUTRIENTS THAT BREATHE LIFE TO YOUR cells

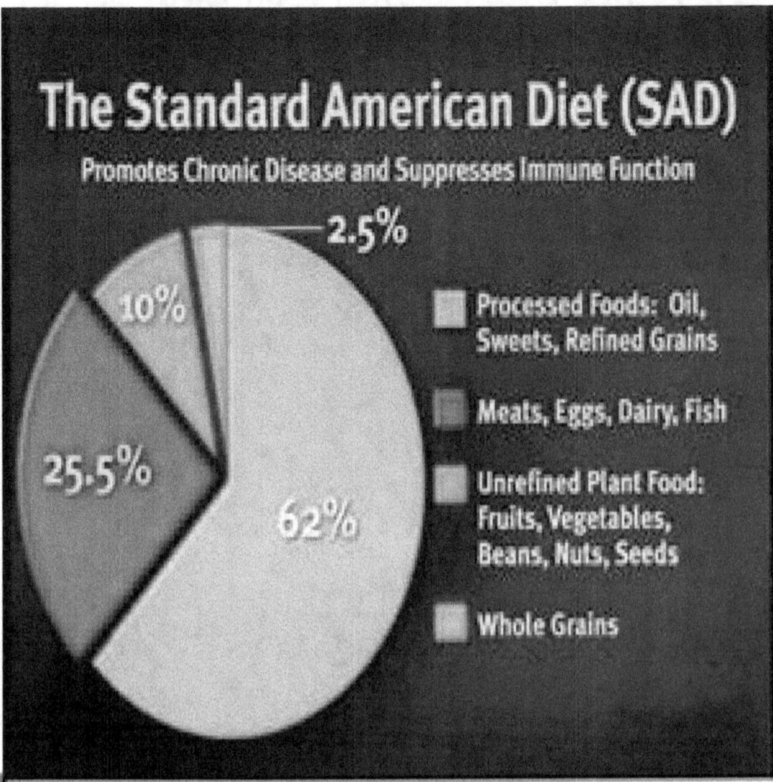

THE NUMBER ONE KILLER IN AMERICA IS FOOD! THE AMERICAN STANDARD
DIET FROM BIRTH. **SUGAR, STARCH, DAIRY (milk, cheese) AND BLOOD**

FROM MEATS WE EAT.

Americans over eat everyday. Learn how to juice;

www.wsaunders.juiceplus.com

AMAZING BODY BENEFITS FROM FRUIT, VEGGIE, BEANS, AND NUTS.
IT IS AWESOME!

GOD's Pharmacy is Amazing

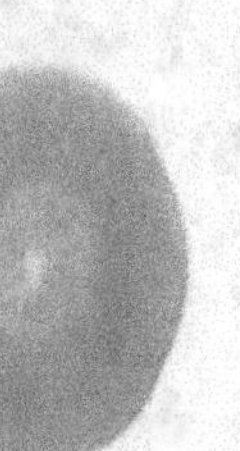

* A sliced carrot looks like a Human eye and it greatly enhances blood flow to the eyes

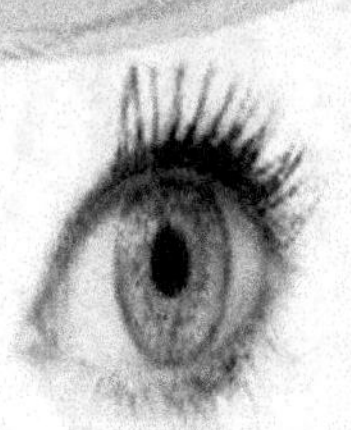

* A tomato has 4 chambers & is red just like the heart. A tomato is loaded with Lycopine that is pure heart & blood food

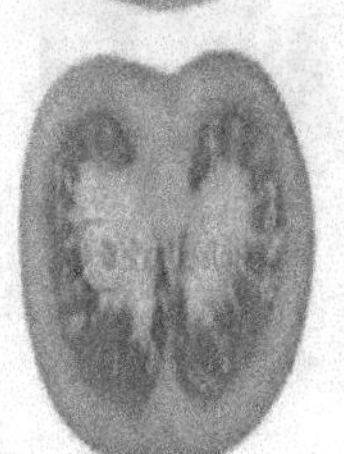

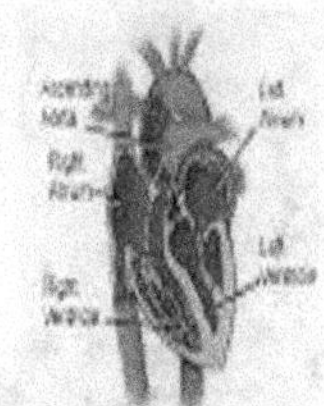

* A walnut looks like the brain and helps develop more than 3 dozen neuro Transmitters to enhance brain functions.

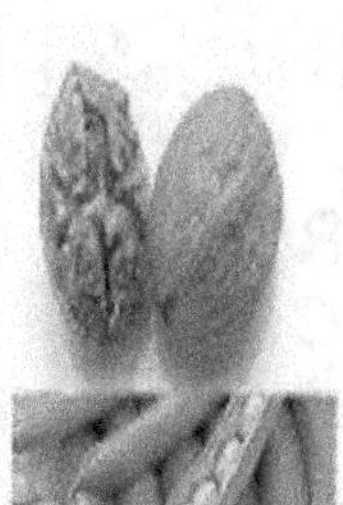

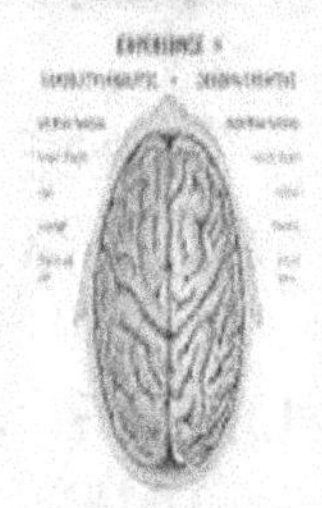

* Beans are kidney shaped and they heal and help maintain kidney functions.

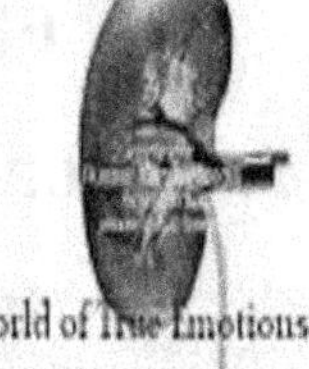

काव्य-संसार - The World of True Emotions

Here Is My Basic Diet Every Day,
Just Giving You Some Ideals

BREAKFAST SUGGESTIONS:

Mixed fruit—(cantaloupe, small bananas, peaches, pears & apples—Whole grain cereal—Old fashioned oatmeal—Flaxseed muffins –Fruit smoothies—Buck wheat pancakes.
Puffed Wheat—Shredded Wheat- and Heart To Heart (Kashi) -Grape Nuts—Raisin Bran— Ralston High Fiber.

YOU CAN HVE YOUR VEGGIES &
FRUITS IN A CAPSULES.

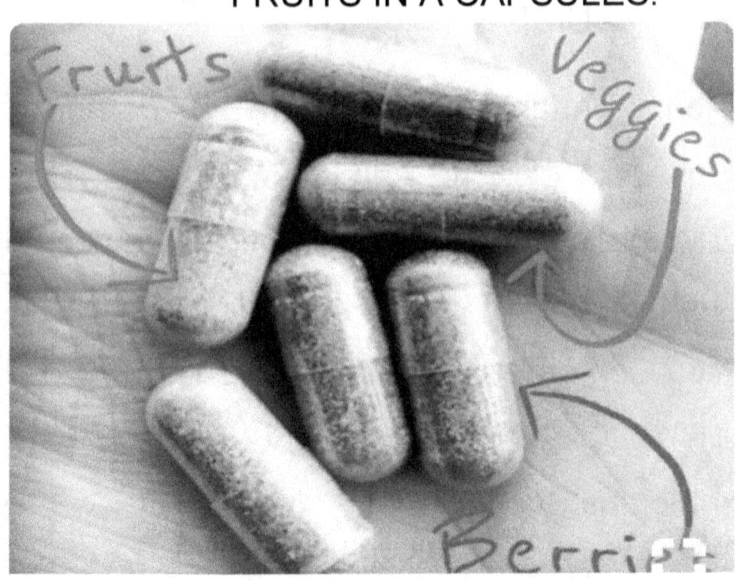

Here Is My Basic Diet Every Day,
Just Giving You Some Ideals

BREAKFAST SUGGESTIONS:

IN A HURRY IN THE MORNING (A vegetable Juice for Energy In The Morning) JUICE RECEIPE:

Need a Juicer or Blender.

Kale, Spinach, Water Cress,

1/2 apple or banana,1 veggie capsule, 1/4 cup of water and blend

If you have pain add: Turmeric & Ginger powder.

FRUIT JUICE:

Apple, Banana, Strawberries, Blue berries, and fruit Capsule & 1/4 water.

If you don't have the fruit capsules you can order them later from me.

You Can order 1 Week Supply: 28.00 Facebook.com/zehira911

4 Months Supply : 44.50 (1.49/day)
www.wsaunders.juiceplus.com

Email: miraclehealing7@yahoo.com

45 SUPER FOODS PLANTS ARE IN
THE
VEGGIE CAPSULES
YOU CAN ALSO TAKE THE CAPSULE
OR OPEN IT AND PUT IT IN YOUR JUICE.

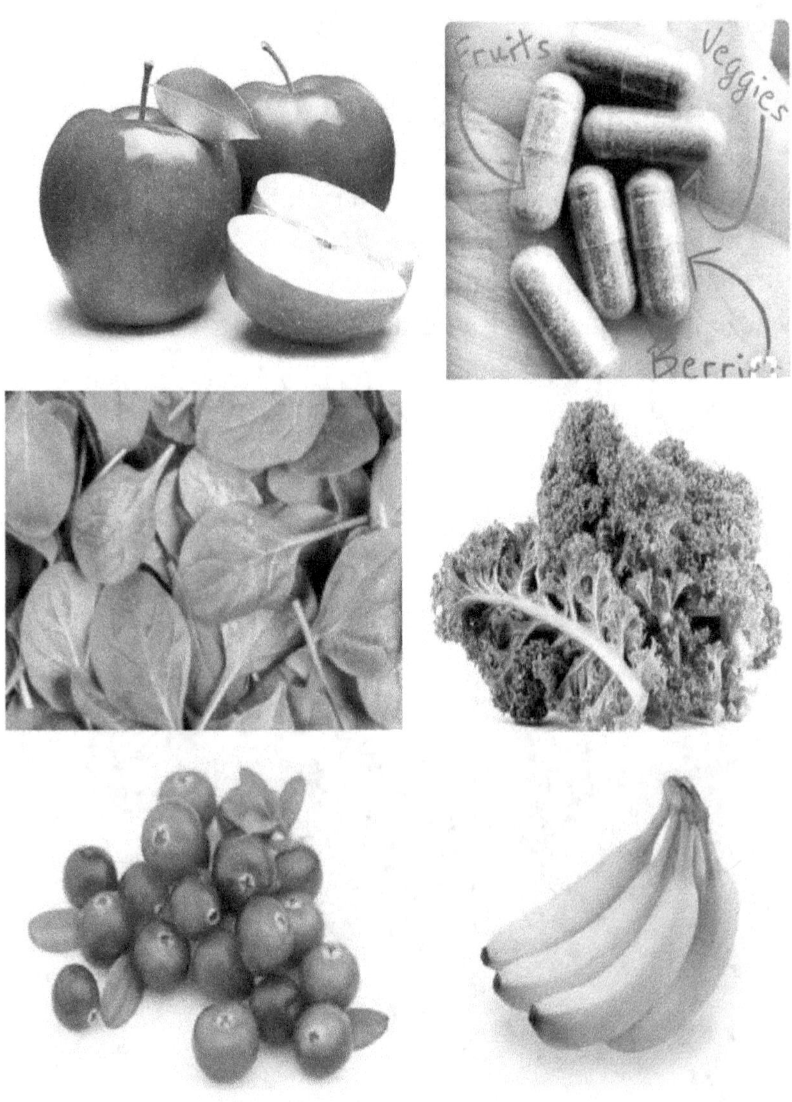

LUNCH OR DINNER
SUGGESTIONS:

Bean soup and stir fried vegetables
Beets, raisins with seeds and
Brown rice and vegetables Salad &
raw vegetables
Stir fry vegetables
Garden salad—vegetable soup
Garden salad wrap—vegetarian chili
Green beans and garlic mashed potato (keep the skin)
Whole wheat pasta tomato sauce and vegetables
Whole grain pasta and vegetables
Raw vegetables
Roasted eggplant, & zucchini wrap

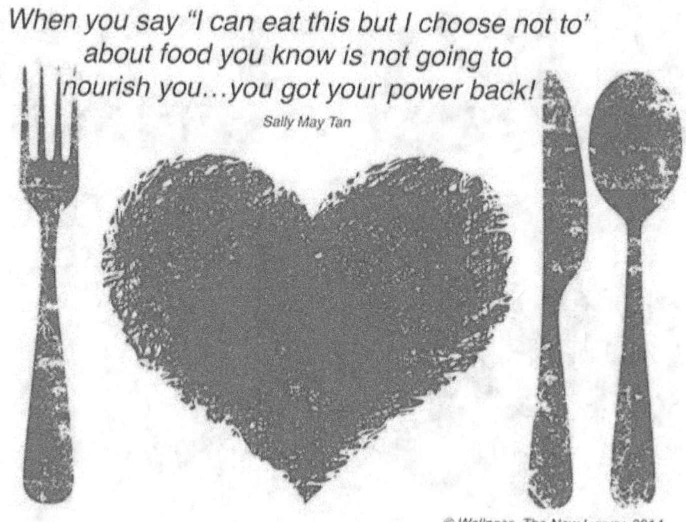

Salty Flavors

Pure Sea Salt
Powdered Granulated Seaweed (Kelp/Dulce/Nori
– has "sea taste")

Sweet Flavors

100% Pure Agave Syrup – (from cactus)
Date Sugar
Grains
Amaranth
Fonio
Kamut
Quinoa
Rye
Spelt
Tef
Wild Rice

Oils
Olive Oil (Do not cook)
Coconut Oil (Do not cook)
Grapeseed Oil
Sesame Oil
Hempseed Oil
Avocado Oil

Additional Resources
*Dr. Sebi has recommended the foods that are
listed here for the reversal of disease for over 30
years. If your favorite food is missing from the
list, our research and results have proven that it
has no nutritional value and may be detrimental
to your health.*

LINDA LARKINS 70 YEARS YOUNG

Her Beauty Secrets Notes I Took From Her Interview On You tube.
To Look And Feel Younger!

Get rid of refined flour and sugar. Eat fruits, nuts and
vegetables, seeds and sprouts.
Drink distilled water, fresh fruit juice, and
vegetable juice.
Exercise, ("I walk three times a week for 20 minutes
at the park and use the machines there.")

Rest, you don't have to do 8 hours, do whatever feels like
rest for you and your body. "I go to bed before 11 and
I wake up after 4 every morning, I lay still and just
meditate and pray in the spirit."

Sunshine, the Doctors recommend 15 minutes a day, to
get natural vitamin C & D. You can stay in the sun
until you think you're had enough, don't get sunburn.

A good mental attitude, think positive as much as
possible. Don't hold on to negative words, let them
go! Be grateful for what you have and don't have, it
will make you feel good.
Love, if you love yourself you can love others, love
people no matter where they are in life and your
neighbors as yourself. (all nations of people of
colors).
Do your own thing, don't want to be someone else you
are one of a kind and special. There is no one on the
earth like you! Grow something indoors or out doors
and watch it grow as you take care of it.

Do something good for someone daily and help where
ever you see the need. It heals the mind and heart.
Giving is very important for staying young. This helps
cleanse your mind, heart and soul. If you know
something that will help fellowman share the
information if it can make them better.

Share, get yourself in the right mold and help each other.
Influence whoever wants information

YOUR NATURAL HEALTH CONSULTANT
(Dr. W. Saunders)
Specialize In Herbs & Nutrition

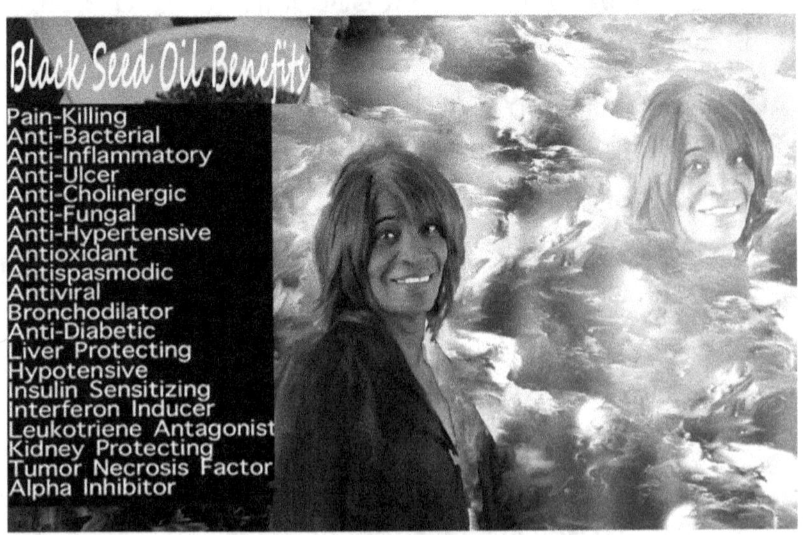

MORINGA TEA & BLACK SEED
CAPSULES CAPSULES

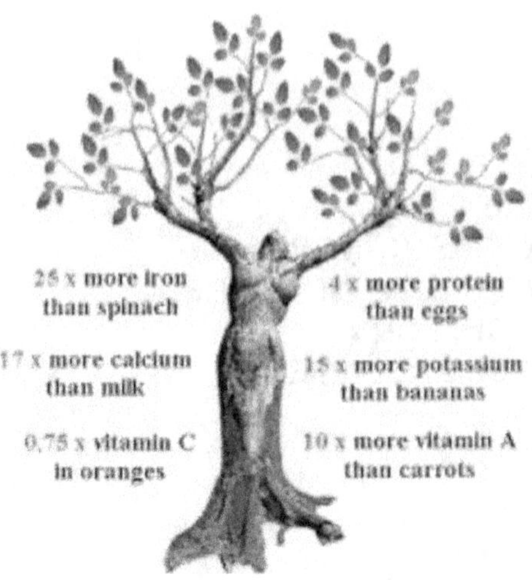

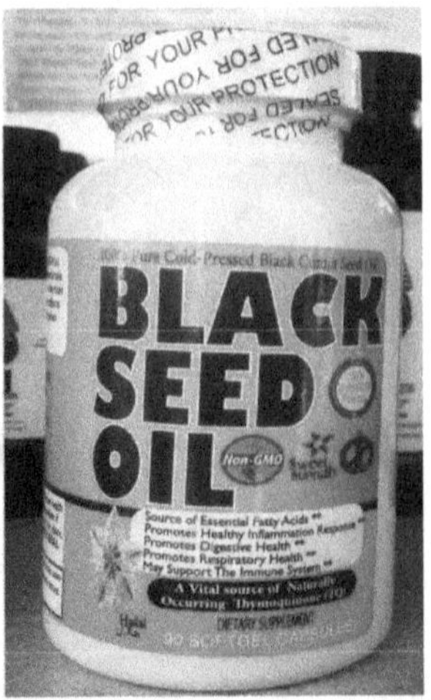

PRAYERS FOR HEALTH

(Genesis 2:9; Ezekiel 47:12; Rev. 22:2)

I BELIEVE THAT YOU FATHER GOD ARE ABLE TO HEAL
THIS _________________________________.
AMEN
ACCORDING TO MY FAITH, TRUST & RELIANCE ON
THE POWER OF THE HOLY SPIRIT INVESTED IN ME.
LET IT BE DONE UNTO ME RIGHT NOW! AMEN

PRAYER FOR HEALTH
(Jeremiah 17:14)

**HEAL ME, O LORD, AND I WILL BE
HEALED; SAVE ME AND I WILL BE SAVED,
FOR YOU ARE
THE ONE I PRAISE !!! AMEN**

We give the medicine, God does
the healing, just believe and trust
your Creator for
healing.

PRAYER FOR WORK
(Job 1:10)

**I HAVE A WONDERFUL WORK, IN A
WONDERFUL WAY, I GIVE WONDERFUL
SERVICE, FOR A
WONDERFUL PAY! AMEN**

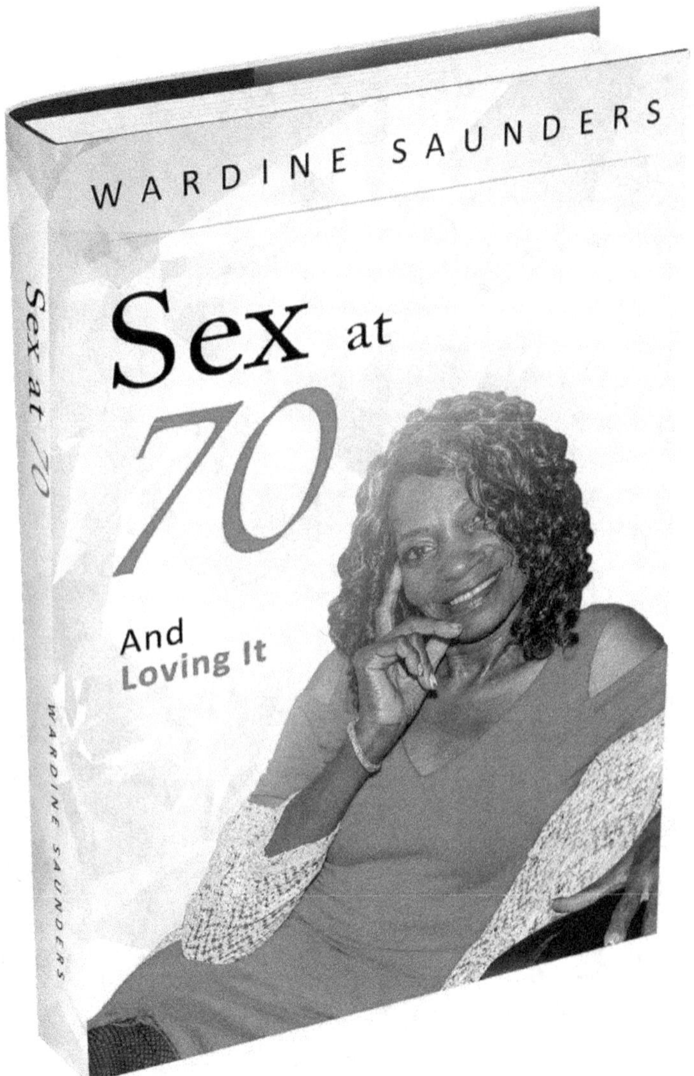

WARDINE SAUNDERS
Sex at
70
And
Loving It
Sex at 70
WARDINE SAUNDERS